Hypertension
Control and Cure
—— *without* ——
Medication

Experience and Testimony
of an Hypertensive
Elderly Man

by Arthur Davis, Jr.

DISCLAIMER
Please Read With Awareness

The information in this book was not written by a medical doctor, professional health care provider, or health professional; this information was written by an elderly man who experienced being a victim, patient, and survivor of Primary Hypertension.

This book is not intended to be a medical guide or give any medical advice concerning any medical conditions.

Please check with your medical doctor or professional health care or health professional to advise you on your medical concerns.

I take or assume no personal responsibility for your medical condition should anyone endeavor to follow any of my writing in this book.

Unless otherwise indicated, Bible quotations are taken from
King James version of the Bible.
Copyright 1909, by Oxford University Press, Inc.

DEDICATION

To:

The Memory of My
Wife; Ola Belle

Mother; Mary
Father; Arthur, Sr.
and
My Sisters
Fannie, Mary, Helen, and Bernice

APPRECIATION

To:

My Children
Vivian*, Vincent, Vickie*, Veronica

My Grand Children
Michael (deceased)
Darius*
LaTanya
Deja
Kimberly*
Willie, Jr.
David
Christopher

My Great Grand Children
Isaiah
Makhi
Kimara
Keondre
Shai

CONTENTS

ACKNOWLEDGMENTS

My Nieces of Encouragement
Gloria Delores Long
Janice Marie Singleton
Shirley Harris

Glory to God

Now unto Him Who is able to keep me from falling and present me faultless before the Presence of His Glory, with exceeding joy, to the only Wise God, my Savior, be Glory and Majesty, Dominion and Power, both now and forever. (Jude 24-25)
Amen

INTRODUCTION

Hypertension Control and Cure without Medication

The information in this book is the personal Experience and Testimony of an Intermediate Elderly man who had to deal with Primary Hypertension, the Type that has no known medical cause or cure.

Realizing that there are millions of people who have this same medical condition gave him, equally, millions of reasons why he needed to write this book.

He will cover four years as a victim, patient, and victor or conqueror of Primary Hypertension. During the last two of the four years, he was on his own using his Alternative Treatment without medication, at the age of 81. And he perfected his Cure at the age of 83.

He starts his book by explaining the True Definition of Hypertension, what *it is not*, and what *it is*. This statement might be considered controversial to some who would define Hypertension as a Disease.

This man accepted his doctor's diagnosis and definition of his medical condition as Primary Hypertension, a Chronic Disease with no known medical cause or cure. He also accepted his doctor's prescribed medication to treat his Hypertension.

After being convinced that Hypertension *is not* a Disease but *is* a Symptom, he implemented his Alternative Treatment, which is an *Eight Step Plan*, without the use of Prescription Medication.

Those who are dealing with the same medical condition may find his experience and testimony interesting, entertaining, enticing, and/or maybe useful.

However, he wishes you the best in obtaining and maintaining your Health and Wellness.

CHAPTER 1

True Definition of Hypertension

Disease or Symptom

Hypertension, also known as High Blood Pressure, has been listed in the catalog of Medical Mysteries, is a very serious Medical Condition that is referred to as *The Silent Killer*, because it claims its victims without, necessarily, showing signs or warnings.

Types of Hypertension

There are two major Types of Hypertension:

1. Primary Hypertension: The Type of Hypertension that is diagnosed as a Chronic Disease with no known medical cause or cure. This Type comprises about 95 percent of the 50,000,000 plus cases of Hypertension.

2. <u>Secondary Hypertension</u>: The Type of Hypertension diagnosed as a Chronic Disease that is closely associated with, or is a part of, some other abnormality within the Body, but there is usually a known medical cause and cure. This Type comprises about 5 percent of the 50,000,000 plus cases of Hypertension.

<u>Process of Defining Hypertension</u>

I am going to explain what I actually experienced and observed in defining Hypertension, what *it is not,* and what *it is.* The characteristics and behavior of Hypertension defines itself as a process:

• <u>Describing</u>, giving details of its characteristics and

• <u>Explaining</u>, clarifying the behavior, purposes or actions.

There are many levels of Blood Pressure, but the definition remains the same. These levels range from very low to very high:

• Low Blood Pressure (LBP): 60/40 to 90/60

- Normal Blood Pressure (NBP), (BP): 100/65 to 130/85

- High Blood Pressure, Hypertension (HBP), (HTN): 140/90 TO 230/140

  Measurements are in millimeters of mercury (mm Hg). The upper number is Systolic, which represents the Blood Pressure when the Heart pumps or expands. The lower number is Diastolic, which represents the Blood Pressure when the Heart muscle relaxes.

Blood Flow In The Process

When the Heart pumps and the Blood flows, this is part of the process of defining Hypertension. The Heart is pumping and pressuring the oxygenated Blood to flow from the left side of the Heart to the upper Body, lung, arms, and head. At the same time, blood also flows to the lower Body, liver, small intestine, kidney, and legs.

After the Blood has made all its deliveries to the different parts of the Body through arteries, small arterioles, and capillaries, the Blood becomes deoxygenated and returns, by way of the veins to the right side of the Heart. The Heart sends this Blood to the lungs to be oxygenated again. Then, the lungs send this Blood to the left side of the Heart to repeat the Systemic Blood circulatory cycle.

During this circulatory cycle, there will always be Pressure within the Heart and Blood circulatory system, along with added Pressure from the walls of the arteries, and other Pressure factors that affect the total Blood Pressure.

<u>Measuring The Process</u>

Let's take a look at how Blood Pressure, so far, has defined itself. When the Blood starts to flow, the Systolic and the Diastolic functions of the Heart show a reading on a Blood Pressure Monitor.

The reading on the Monitor will change when any of the many factors that affect the Pressure changes; when the Blood Pressure reading is high, this means that there is something within the circulatory system or influential environment that is increasing the resistance to the flow of Blood.

Sensitivity And Reactions

Please notice, the High Blood Pressure reading is not the Cause, within itself, for the High Blood Pressure. The High Blood Pressure reading is recording or registering the results of something that causes an increase in Blood Pressure, and *not* the Blood Pressure itself.

High Blood Pressure or Hypertension, so far, is defining itself. it has been responsive to the Causes for the changes in Blood flow, and these changes are recorded or registered on the Blood Pressure Monitor as Systolic and Diastolic functions.

Personal Encounter

My doctor could not find a Cause for my High Blood Pressure , or Hypertension. This put my doctor in a precarious situation of having to make a diagnosis of a medical condition that is listed with some of the other Medical Mysteries; define and classify this Condition as a Chronic Disease, Primary Hypertension; and lastly, and most seriously, having to prescribe Medication for an unknown Cause.

Making A Point With Body Temperature

My doctor took my temperature and the thermometer read 102 degrees, My doctor examined me, found the Cause for the high temperature, gave me some information and a prescription, and I was on my way.

The temperature was not my medical condition; my temperature was a Symptom of my medical condition. The thermometer recorded or registered the temperature, the Symptom.

Making A Point With Secondary Hypertension

My doctor took my Blood Pressure. The Blood Pressure Monitor reading was very high, somewhere around 200/110. After ten minutes, my Pressure was still very high, My doctor did an examination but could not find any Cause for my High Pressure. I was given a prescription for the High Blood Pressure, some information, an appointment to return in one week, and I was on my way.

I returned on the day of my appointment. My doctor did another examination and discovered that I had a Kidney infection, which was the Primary Disease and the Primary Cause. My Secondary Hypertension was my Secondary Disease and the Secondary Cause.

I was given several Prescriptions to treat both Conditions, some information, and I was on my way.

After about six months, the Kidney infection was cured and my Blood Pressure was down to normal.

The Disease was an infected Kidney; but since the Hypertension seemed to have been related to the Primary Disease, Hypertension becomes the Secondary Disease and, consequently, Secondary Hypertension.

<u>Making A Point With Primary Hypertension</u>

My doctor took my Blood Pressure. The Blood Pressure Monitor reading was very high, somewhere around 200/110. After ten minutes, my Pressure was still very high. My doctor did an examination but could not find any Cause for my High Pressure; I was given a prescription for the High Blood Pressure, some information, an appointment to return in one week, and I was on my way.

I returned on the day of my appointment. my Blood Pressure was down some, but still too high. My doctor did another examination and ran some tests, explained some things, advised me to continue taking the medication, gave me my next appointment date, and I was on my way.

On my appointment date, I was back to my doctor's office to receive the results from the tests. Nothing was found to cause my Hypertension, so the doctor's final diagnosis was a Chronic Disease, called Primary Hypertension no other Medical Cause for my Hypertension could be diagnosed.

Remember that Primary Hypertension has no known Medical Cause or Cure. This is a challenge for any doctor to have to treat a patient with this Medical Condition that is considered to be a Chronic Disease, has no known medical Cause or Cure and must be treated with trial medication with only tentative results expected.

Doctor's Final Words

The words from my doctor to me, "To keep your Hypertension under control, you will have to take medication the rest of your life."

Solving The Medical Mystery Of The Silent Killer

History records as far back as 2600 BC report that there was a Disease called Hard Pulse Disease, also known as Hypertension. We are looking at a time frame of nearly 3000 years and Hypertension is still being diagnosed and defined as a Chronic Disease.

It is extremely important and absolutely necessary, that Hypertension be accurately and faithfully defined.

Through the efforts of Medical Science, Doctors, and other Medical Professionals, we have witnessed tremendous changes and improvements in Treatment for Hypertension.

However, it seems that in solving the case of the Medical Mystery of Hypertension, The Silent Killer, defining or positively identifying the Killer , Hypertension, should be elementary.

What *It Is Not* But What *It Is*

Hypertension *is no*t a Disease. A Disease is a medical condition that has a Cause, an Effect, and a Symptom. All Diseases have a Cause, an Effect, and a Symptom. In the laws of Cause and Effect, Hypertension does not have a Cause an Effect, and a Symptom, because it is the Symptom.

Hypertension *is* a Symptom. A Symptom is a sign or an indicator of an abnormal Condition, a Disease, or an Illness that can be: Physical, Mental or Spiritual. These signs or indicators can be displayed in many different ways: Blood Pressure Monitors, registers, oscilloscopes, gauges, and so forth.

My Health and Wellness

Is
My Responsibility

To Know As Much About <u>Hypertension</u>
As I Can

CHAPTER 2

Hypertension Causes

<u>Secondary Hypertension Has A Known Cause, Maybe</u>

Secondary Hypertension Causes are directly related to disorders or diseases in some specific parts of the Body, Mind, Soul, or Spirit. This Type, Secondary Hypertension, may be considered as a Misnomer for two reasons:

1. Medical Professionals define Hypertension as a Disease when in fact, it is a Symptom of a Disease or Illness.
2. My Medical Condition, Primary Hypertension is a Primary Disease because no Cause was found. If a Cause had been found, then my Medical Condition would have been Secondary Hypertension, a Secondary Disease. There is some doubt if Secondary Hypertension is diagnosed correctly.

All of Me

In my living-the-experience in dealing with Hypertension, it is reasonable, to me, to expect that any activity of the Body, Mind, Soul, or Spirit can affect the Blood Pressure. Unfortunately, Medical Professionals deal with only half of the total person, Body and Mind, but there are the Soul and the Spirit that should also be addressed.

Common Ground

Secondary Hypertension finds support when some Disease diagnosed in a few of the areas of common Causes are:

- Heart: The Heart can experience many disorders or Diseases that are causes for Secondary Hypertension, cardiovascular Disease, heart attack and coronary artery Disease.

- Arteries and blood vessels: Arteries and Blood vessels can become damaged, clogged or Diseased.

- Kidneys: Kidneys can experience tumors, failure, blocked or narrowed renal artery.

Those are some common cases of known Diseases and Causes in dealing with Secondary Hypertension, which make up about 5 percent of the total cases of all Hypertension.

If the Diseases and Causes are found in the Heart, Arteries or Kidney, Secondary Hypertension is still Diagnosed as the secondary Disease.

<u>Primary Hypertension Has an Unknown Cause, Maybe</u>

The other basic type of High Blood Pressure is Primary Hypertension, which has no medically-known Cause or Cure, and makes up the other 95 percent of the total cases of Hypertension.

Medical Science has followed and measured our Blood flow through the entire circulatory system to all our organs, to all our extremities, to every area of our Body searching for the Cause or Causes for Primary Hypertension, but with no success.

My doctors admitted to me that they did not know the Cause for my Type of Hypertension, which was Primary Hypertension, and I would have to take medication the rest of my life to possibly maintain my Blood Pressure within a safe range.

Final Decision

So I had to decide on an Alternative to Conventional Medicine to deal with this Mysterious Medical Condition with an unknown Medical Cause or Cure, and indeed I did.

My Health and Wellness

Is
My Responsibility

To Get The **Best Diagnosis**
That I Can

CHAPTER 3

Hypertension Effects

<u>No Favorites</u>

The Hypertension Effects can be a threat to human life; harm, damage, and suffering can be overwhelming. Even death can be the result of the Hypertension Effects. No part of the human Body is immune from Hypertension Effects, from head to feet.

We are subject to this mysterious, invisible, quiet, malicious, and deadly Entity, Hypertension, that is usually identified with the Silent Killer as a Metaphor.

<u>Looking For A Sign</u>

It is generally stated that Hypertension usually starts with no Sign or Symptom to alert its victim of its presence. But in fact,

Hypertension *is* the *Sign* or *Symptom* that something abnormal is happening in the Body.

Even after I am aware of experiencing some abnormal condition, the Effects may not be correctly diagnosed. If Secondary Hypertension is the Type that has been diagnosed, then the medical condition has been traced to a Cause, other than Hypertension, that can be treated to correct or eliminate the abnormal condition or Disease. Some common areas where the Hypertension Effects are experienced:

- Brain, needs a continuing supply of nourishing Blood to function properly for survival. Hypertension Effects are Blood clots forming in the arteries leading to the Brain that can cause a stroke, or a Blood vessel wall to burst, which can cause bleeding in the Brain.

- Kidneys filter excess fluid and waste from the Blood, which depends on healthy, regulated Blood Pressure.

Tit for Tat

The Kidneys say to Blood Pressure, "If you keep your Blood Pressure down, I will keep your Blood clean".

The Blood Pressure says to the Kidneys, "If you keep your Kidneys healthy, I will keep my Blood Pressure down".

The Faithful Heart

The heart pumps Blood through our circulatory system to every nook and cranny of our Body, every moment of our life. What a Heart!

Some common Hypertension Effects:

- Coronary Artery Disease,

- Congestive Heart failure and

- Diastolic Dysfunction.

As Many Effects As Causes

There are probably as many Hypertension Effects as there are known and unknown Hypertension Causes.

However, I am not able to share any personal experience with Hypertension Effects, because I do not know what they were. I also didn't know my Hypertension Cause; if the Cause is unknown, then the Effect is unknown, Cause and Effect..

Known Effects Not Necessary

My Alternative Treatment is all inclusive. In my case, it did not matter whether the Causes and Effects were known or unknown, my Treatment was able to Control and Cure my Medical Condition, Medically diagnosed as Primary Hypertension.

My Health and Wellness

Is

My Responsibility

To Know As Much About **Hypertension Effects** As I Can

CHAPTER 4

Hypertension Test

<u>What A Test Can Reveal</u>

In 2006, an important Test in my life was a High Blood Pressure or Hypertension Test. That Test revealed that I had a Medical Condition with an unknown Medical Cause and an unknown Cure, Primary Hypertension, also known as **The Silent Killer** .

<u>Wake Up Call</u>

After realizing the Life-Threatening danger that complements Hypertension, High Blood Pressure, I had even more reasons to fear this Killer, because of some of the characteristics of Hypertension:

- No signs

- No symptoms

- Silent

- Insidious

- Malicious

- Deadly

Those characteristics are not to be ignored, especially when it's my life that could be the target.

How Testing Got Started

Testing or measuring Blood Pressure was recorded back in 1733, by the Reverend Stephen Hales, a British veterinarian. He took a horse and inserted a brass pipe into an artery; this pipe was connected to a glass tube. Hales observed the rising Blood in the pipe and concluded that it must be due to a Pressure in the Blood.

In 1896, Scipione Riva-Rocci developed the mercury sphygmomanometer. This design was the prototype of the modern mercury sphygmomanometer.

In 1905, Nikolai Korotkoff was the first to observe the sounds at certain points in the inflation and deflation of the cuff. The sounds were caused by the abnormal passage of Blood through the artery corresponding to the Systolic and Diastolic Blood Pressures while using a stethoscope to listen for the sounds of Blood flowing through the artery.

Twenty-First Century Testing

Doctors use the following instruments in their office to measure the patient's Blood Pressure:

1. Anerold Sphygmomanometer, a device used to measure Blood Pressure comprising an inflatable cuff to restrict Blood flow and a mercury or mechanical manometer to measure the Pressure; this was used in conjunction with a means to determine at what pressure the Blood flow is just starting, and at what pressure it is restricted.
2. Manual Sphygmomanometers are used with a stethoscope.

The readings from these instruments showing or indicating the patient's Blood Pressure will assist the doctor in arriving at a diagnosis of the patient's medical condition.

The accuracy of these instruments and the interpretation of the readings are essential to the doctor's correct diagnosis. The correct diagnosis is essential in order that the patient receive the correct and best treatment.

It all started with the Testing. The purpose was to determine if Hypertension, The Silent Killer was lurking within my Body.

In-Home Testing

Medical Technology has made it possible for any household to be able to Test for Hypertension right in the home. There are Blood Pressure Monitors that come in different types, including Finger, Wrist, and Cuff. I will talk more about this medical instrument in the chapter on Monitors.

You might want to think about getting Tested for Hypertension. Getting a well-intentioned Test might reveal an ill-Health medical condition.

My Health and Wellness

Is
My Responsibility

To Get The **Best Test** That I Can

CHAPTER 5

Hypertension Treatment Start Up

Tested, Now Treat

In the previous chapter, my doctor completed all the Testing, arrived at a diagnosis, and is now ready to start my Primary Hypertension Treatment. Remember, this type Hypertension has no known Medical Cause or Cure. So this is a most challenging and perplexing responsibility for both the doctor and the patient in the Treatment for this Medical Condition.

Did What I Had To Do

After learning about some of the characteristics of Hypertension, I discovered some very bad things, that even Death is related to this Medical Condition. I had no other choice but to go along with my doctor's Treatment

27

Program, which consisted, primarily, of Medication. My doctor informed me that I would probably have to take Medication the rest of my life, just to try and keep my Blood Pressure within a safe range.

For about two years, I followed my doctor's Treatment Program, agreeing to take the Prescription Medication.

After two years on my doctor's Treatment Program, I realized that I had subjected my body to, possibly, many adverse known and unknown side effects from the Medication that I had been taking for a Medical Condition with an unknown Medical Cause or Cure.

Time For Change

Throughout this book, I talk about Personal Responsibility by using my personal living experiences. My understanding of the True Definition of Hypertension is important to me in deciding to follow my Alternative Treatment.

I was definitely sure that I, the patient, not the doctor, had to assume my Responsibility for my Health.

I decided this was the time for me to choose an Alternative Approach rather than Conventional Medicine. My decision was, indeed, challenging and perplexing. However, I respectfully went against my doctor's advice, and discontinued the use of Prescription Medication.

There is no Medical training or experience in my background. But in making the decision to follow my Alternative Approach, I knew having a Medical background was not necessary.

My Eight-Point Plan:

1. Diet/Menu, I consider all my Foods, inclusive, to be my Menu, including herbal spices and supplements.
2. Water: I use two types, one for drinking and the other for cooking .
3. Air: I deal with indoor environment as an internal earth and atmosphere.
4. Exercise: I Exercise using my creative techniques and routines, without equipment.
5. Monitoring: I am able to monitor all of my Anatomy's Blood Pressure -related activities.

6. Courage: Courage is absolutely necessary in both the Physical and the Spiritual Aspects or Activities of my Life.
7. Faith: Without Faith, it is impossible to please God, and It is the Life Blood of my Spiritual Life.
8. Spirituality: Spirituality is relating to God, Christ, the Holy Spirit, Word of God, Soul, and Body.

This Plan worked for me to Control and Cure my Primary Hypertension, to maintain my Control and Cure. I continue to use this Plan, but with less activity in some areas.

My Health and Wellness

Is
My Responsibility

To Receive The **Best Treatment**
That I Can

CHAPTER 6

Hypertension Treatment – Diet/Menu

I Am What I Eat

Actually, I am *more* than what I eat. You might recall that old adage, "we are what we eat," or "you are what you eat." That is not the whole truth. We are only part of what we eat.

The truth is, "what I eat is only a part of what I am," that is my own adage, or axiom. I will use what I am as a focal point when bringing all parts together that is relative to what I am.

In the process of determining what I am, I will look at the basic, essential requirements that sustain my Natural or Physical Life:

- **Food** that I Eat sustains my Physical Life, only if I have Water to Drink and Air to Breath;

- **Water** that I Drink sustains my Physical Life, only if I have Food to Eat and Air to Breath

- **Air** that I Breath sustains my Physical Life, only if I have Food to Eat and Water to Drink. I see that my Physical life cannot be sustained by any *one* without the *other two*. It might seem that all are in place and *what I am* is complete. However, not quite; there is a fourth part.

- **Spirituality** that I Believe sustains my Spiritual Life and Physical Life, and is indispensable if I am to be all that I was created to be. This includes *what I am* and, most of all, *who I am*. This essential fourth part sustains my Spiritual Life through the Word of God being relative to my Body, Mind, Soul, and Spirit; and it also sustains and enhances my Physical Life. I'll touch much more on my Spiritual Life in chapter 12.

The Importance of the Natural or Physical and the Spiritual

What I am and *who I am* were from the time of Creation, and I realize the importance of being aware of this status because:

God *made* man from the dust of the earth; but He *created* man from His Spirit. Remem-

ber, the part of man He *made* is (*what I am*) Natural, Physical, Earthy, and the part of man He created is (*who I am*) Spiritual, in His Likeness. (Genesis 1:26-27; 2:7)

Diet or Menu

In changing *what I am*, I will start with changing my Menu. I choose to use *Menu* rather than *Diet* because there are more than 250 Diets out there and I don't want my Menu to get lost in the mix;. Other reasons for my choice to use *Menu*:

• Diet seems to suggest Duty, Regimentation, Restriction, Limitation, Loss of Freedom, and Lack of Excitement. All of these things are a little like *laws.*

• Menu seems to suggest Privilege, Choice, Anticipation, Excitement, Freedom, and Joy. All of these things are a little like Grace.

Originating the Food Chain

Farmers have to make sure the *seeds* they plant are good, quality *seeds,* not necessarily Genetically-Modified Organisms (GMO).

Hopefully, they are not growing Genetically-Modified Food. If this Type of Food gets to the Market Place, it might be the only food available for our Selection. Another concern the Public might have about the *seeds is that* some of the *seeds* may be classified as *Terminator Genes* or *Suicide Seeds,* which alters the DNA of the *seeds,* and is good for only one generation.

The Farmers producing our meats are as concerned about providing Good Food from the Live Stock as from the Vegetables and Fruits. The Farmers have factors to contend with that could challenge the quality of their Crops and Live Stock:

- Weather can be a Friend or Foe.

- Harvesting must be done properly, and in a timely manner, to maintain the quality of the products.

- Storage is critical, as to the manner and area, in keeping the products fresh and undamaged.

The Fishermen are faced with a growing challenge that constantly threatens the quality of our seafood. The lakes, rivers, and oceans, the only environments for fish and other seafood, are being Polluted with chemicals and waste. Some major concerns for the Fishermen are the many Pollutants that affect their products, as well as Harvesting and Storage.

The Food Manufacturers and Corporations cover most of the spectrum of the food industry. They work in conjunction with Farmers and Fishermen and have to meet safety and nutrition regulations of the Food and Drug Administration (FDA) and U.S. Department of Agriculture (USDA.

In some areas of our Food Chain, the Corporations may have an agenda to completely eliminate what few Farmers and Fishermen still exist; their days are already numbered.

Quality of Our Food

The Entities that produce, harvest, store, and deliver our Foods should be seriously concerned about the quality of our Food.

- *Good Food* contains all or most of its respective, original nourishing substances that were provided organically by nature to help keep the human body healthy, if ingested in the proper manner.

- *Bad Food* contains little of its respective, original nourishing substances that were provided organically by nature and may not be much help in keeping the human body healthy, even when ingested in the proper manner.

- *Deadly Food* may contain very little of its respective, original nourishing substances that were provided organically by nature, but contains substances that are harmful, even Life-Threatening, to the human Body, if ingested in any manner.

Using Our Senses in Testing Food

The Food Chain starts at *seed time* and the quality of our Food, whether Good, Bad, or Deadly, can start at *seed time* or any other time or place thereafter.

The public is concerned about the quality of the Food when it is reaches the market place; this is when we use our senses to test the quality of the Food:

- **<u>Looks Good</u>**, physical appearance that is pleasing to the eyes.

- **<u>Feels Good</u>**: Touch that passes one of the tests for quality.

- **<u>Smells Good;</u>**. A distinctive quality detected by smell.

- **<u>Tastes Good</u>**: This may not always be accommodated in the market place. Taste pertains to sweetness, saltiness, bitterness, or sourness.

<u>Personal Responsibility for Quality of Food</u>

After I have made my Food Selection at the market place, assuming that I have made a good quality Selection, it is my Responsibility to maintain that quality until it reaches the dinner table.

There are two basic activities and Food Links that are the Responsibilities of the consumer in the home in order to prevent Good Food from being adversely affected:

1. Storage can be a major concern before and after Preparation. Use quality containers.
2. Preparation is the last link and requires a lot of the basic things, especially cooking habits and seasoning to suit the taste, which can be good, or not so good, for the Health.

My Kitchen and All Therein

A lot goes on in the kitchen that can have a tremendous impact on my Health. I try to cover all of what happens, how it happens, and why it happens for the sake of Health.

The kitchen is where I make sure that the one-fourth (1/4) part of *what I am* contributes the best it can in harmony with the other three (3) parts.

Pots And Pans

This is a list of my kitchen Utensils that are normally used in Food Preparation for a Vegetarian. I was a Pesco (no seafood in the Menu) Vegetarian when I compiled this kitchen inventory:

- 1 Granite ware Pot, 7 quart
- 1 Crock Pot, Medium size
- 1 Sauce Pan, 3 quart, Stainless Steel
- 1 Cutting Board, White Polyethylene, 7 X 10 inches with 4 inch handle
- 1 Large Spoon Non Stick, Long Handle, High Heat Resistant 400F
- 1 Set Of Spatulas, Rubber
- 1 Set Of Spatulas, Plastic
- 1 Strainer, Fine Mesh, 6 Inches
- 2 Measuring Cups, Glass 1 Cup and 4 Cups
- 1 Set Of Measuring Spoon, Plastic
- 1 Set Of Measuring Scoops, Plastic
- 1 Set Of Funnels, Plastic
- 1 Can Opener, Manual
- 1 Salad Spinner

- 1 Mortar and Pestle Set

- 4 Sets of Food Containers, Vacuum, Plastic, Very important items for Storage of vegetables and fruits before and after Preparation.

- 1 Pack of Skewers Sticks, Bamboo, 12 inches

- 1 Knife Sharpener

- 1 Set of Stainless Steel Drinking Straws, convenient for sipping Water.

- Knives, Forks, Spoons, Plates, Saucers, Cups, Bowls, Glasses

Appliances:
- 1 Rice Cooker and Steamer
- 1 Crock Pot, Slow and Medium Cooker
- 1 Oven, Counter Top
- 1 Vegetable And Fruit Juicer
- 1 Blender, Counter Top
- 1 Blender, Hand
- 1 Food Chopper, Small
- 1 Spice And Nut Grinder

- 1 Can Opener
- 1 Kitchen Scale, Digital, 6 Lb. Max
- 1 Water Filter, Counter Top
- 1 Microwave Oven

I have not used my Microwave Oven since 2006. In 1976, the Soviet Union issued a ban on the use of the Microwave Oven. Check out the article *Microwave Oven: The Hidden Hazards* here: http://curezone.com/foods/microwave_oven_risk.asp

Menu, Choices, and Preparations:

The following is a list of my Foods and Preparations as a Vegetarian:

Bread

In the Old Testament, Bread, or Manna *from Heaven* , Physically sustained the people of Israel. Bread, Manna, was used as Food for Life in the wilderness for 40 years.

Before the twentieth-century BC, the Egyptians baked Bread. All along the way, Bread has been a Staple Food, and is known *as the Staff of Life.*

Both the Natural/Physical Bread and Spiritual Bread are necessary to sustain the health of mankind.

- Natural/Physical Bread *sustains* Physical Life. My personal choice of Physical Bread is a flourless, whole-grain bread made from sprouted wheat, barley, millet, lentils, soybeans, and spelt, organic certified grain.

- Spiritual Bread *gives,* and also *sustains,* both Spiritual Life and Physical Life; my personal choice of Spiritual Bread is the Word of God.

Cereals

- Brown Rice, Long Grain, Organic Certified
- Rolled Oaks, Gluten Free
- Hot Cereal, Gluten Free

Fruits

- Apples
- Bananas

- Cantaloupe
- Cherries
- Dates
- Figs
- Grapefruits
- Grapes
- Honey - Raw
- Honeydew Melon
- Mangoes
- Oranges
- Pears
- Pine Apples
- Raisin

Vegetables
- Beans, Green
- Beets
- Broccoli
- Brussels Spouts
- Cabbage, Green And Red

- Cauliflower
- Carrots
- Collard Greens
- Garlic
- Onion, Red
- Potatoes
- Potatoes, Yams
- Rutabaga
- Squash
- Turnips

Cooking Method: Steam Only, all Vegetables.

Dried Beans

- Butter Beans
- Great Northern
- Kidney
- Lima
- Navy
- Pinto
- Red

Cooking Method: Crock Pot Only, all dried Beans.

Seafood

The following Seafood is no longer included on my Menu:

- Salmon
- Sardine
- Tuna

Cooking Method for Salmon: Bake Only

Oils

- Coconut Oil, Extra Virgin
- Olive Oil, Extra Virgin

Coconut Oil, Use Only For Baking and Frying, I never Fry!

Herbs and Spices

- Alfalfa Powder
- Basil Leaf Flakes
- Cayenne Pepper Powder
- Cinnamon Powder

- Clove Powder
- Flax Seed Powder
- Garlic Powder
- Rosemary Powder
- Sea Salt, Celtic
- Vinegar, Apple Cider

Supplements

- B6, 100 MG Capsules
- B12, 1 MG Lozenges
- CoQ10, 100 MG Liquid
- Calcium, Magnesium with Vitamin D, 100 MG Calcium, 500 MG Magnesium, 400 IU Vitamin D Capsules
- Honey, Raw
- Lecithin Granules, for use in my Protein Drink. also sprinkle over my Food.
- Soy Protein Powder, for use in my Protein Drink.
- Chlorella Powder, for use in my Protein Drink, please check out this product.

- Spirulina Powder, for use in my protein Drink, please check out this product.

Seeds And Nuts

- Almonds: Good to make nut butter with using a Seed and Nut Grinder. I recommend this nut butter for Senior Citizens.

- Cashews: Also good to make nut butter

- Pecans: Make good nut butter

- Pumpkin Seeds/Pepitas: I powder them in a Nut Grinder and use in my Protein Drink.

- Sesame Seeds: I powder them in a Nut Grinder and sprinkle over my Food.

- Sunflower Seeds: I powder them in a Nut Grinder and use in my Protein Drink.

- Walnuts

Reasons For Eating

There are as many reasons for eating as there are people. But when you really look at it, there are basically only two reasons why we eat, pretty much like marriage: for **better** or for **worse**.

Now that the Pantry is closed, remember *what I am* is only a part of *what I eat*. But that one-fourth part can carry a lot of weight, **for better or for worse**.

Living Is A Battle

On a national level, when we go to war against a nation, two of our major concerns are:

- Manpower and

- Health of that Manpower. Only those in Good Health will be selected to serve as our soldiers.

On a personal level, we are constantly at war against the forces that are a threat to our Health and even Our Life. To be able to win the battle against those forces, that have no sympathy for the weak and sickly, then we have to be in Good Health.

Everyday, I am in a battle for the right to live, and I have to fight regardless of the condition of my Health.

One of the essentials for Good Health is Good Food, which offers two Good Reasons why I should not settle for less:

1. If I am sick, Good Food will help promote my Healing,
2. If I am well, Good Food will help maintain my Wellness.

Conclusion of What I Eat

You now know how I identify and properly Select, Store, and Prepare Good Food for Consumption from my Diet/Menu of Choice. I have shared with you how *I am what I eat* is one part of *what I am.*

My Health and Wellness

Is

My Responsibility

To Eat The **Best Food** That I Can

CHAPTER 7

Hypertension Treatment – Water

Pure Beyond Measure

In the beginning was Water, and Water was Pure and Good. After Water, there was Light. After Light, Earth appeared. And after Earth appeared, Food appeared. After Food appeared, all living Creatures appeared: Creatures in the Waters, Creatures on Earth, and Creatures in the Air.

There was one Creature on Earth, a Special Species called Man, that was given the Ability and Authority to control all the other Creatures on Earth, above Earth, and below Earth. Man was also given the Responsiblity to maintain all of the Pure Water, which was divided into four main rivers of Pure Water to flow throughout Earth as directed by Nature.

This Special Species, Man, was *not* given the Authority to *control* the Pure Water, but was given the Responsibility to Protect and Preserve the Integrity of the Pure Water.

All Creation and Creatures had free access to Life-Sustaining Pure Water.

Leave It To Man

But then it happened. The *one* Creature, the Special Species, Man, along with his Helpmate, decided to disobey God. Now this was no small *matter*.

We are going to have to take some time to take a really good look at the impact and consequences of this Man and this Woman's one single Act of Disobedience This Act changed the Course of everything that God had Created, all Creation. The full impact and consequences of this Act can be explained only by God!

One thing we do know is that Earth was Cursed and Pure Water lost its Purity. Not only Water, but everything on Earth was Polluted and Contaminated, a whole Planet and its Inhabitants subject to Sicknesses, Suffering, and Death.

Making the Most of It

In the meantime, this present generation of Creatures and Creation is forced to accept the Impure Water left by our Forefathers. To make matters worse, Man is now Polluting and Contaminating our Planet at a faster rate than ever.

All Creation is at the mercy of Man who seems to have very little concern for the Health or Wellness of the environment for Creatures, Creation, or himself.

Many Suffer, Few Profit

Since Water Pollution has become a worldwide problem, a worldwide demand for clean Water has created a Profit Motivation comparable to that of Oil.

Water is now referred to as *Blue Gold*; worldwide Water Prospectors are in desperate search for the Blue Gold and we can see their products, bottled Water, practically everywhere in the world.

These Water Prospectors are trying to gain more influence in our lives by Privatization of our local Water utilities. They are also pumping Water from our lakes and rivers and selling it back to us in bottles.

Definition of Water

The Definition of Water in its Pure state, at the time of Creation, can only be a Conjecture or Theory because there were no Human means for content or quality evaluation.

After the Fall, all of Earth was Cursed. The Waters that flowed in the Rivers were Impure because of the Curse. The four Rivers (the Pison, Gihon, Hiddekel, and Euphrates) that supply Water to all Creatures and Creation, are now flowing in unclean vessels.

The closest we can come to obtaining Pure Water is probably through Nature's Filtering Systems, such as Clouds and Artesian Wells.

When taking a closer look at Water, we see:

- Water is a liquid substance that was in existence before Creation.

- All Life in Creation came from Pure Water, except Man, who came from the Earth.

- Life is sustained by Water.

- Water is colorless and clear.

- Water consists of, basically, two chemical elements: two Atoms of Hydrogen and one Atom of Oxygen.

- Water is part of the Physical Life-Sustaining trinity: Food, Water, and Air.

Sources of Drinking Water

- Surface Water supply is on or above ground.

- Ground Water supply is below ground level.

- Surface/Ground Water supply is from both sources.

Types of Drinking Water

- Tap Water is from faucets.

- Distilled Water is bottled from surface Water.

- Mineral Water is bottled from underground Water.

- Spring Water is bottled from underground Water.

- Filtered Water is bottled from surface Water and countertop filtering.

Making Water Safe

Nature is most Merciful and Gracious to Destructive and Ungrateful Mankind. It still provides Water Filtering Systems to make Man-Polluted Water safe enough for Man to drink and use.

Working with Nature, the Safe Drinking Water Act, SDWA, and Environmental Protection Act, EPA, set standards to ensure the quality of the drinking Water and oversee the states, localities, and suppliers who implement those standards. Law Enforcement also requires many actions to protect the drinking Water Sources including rivers, lakes, reservoirs, springs, and groundwater wells.

The Qualities of Water:

- Good/Safe Water: Water that contains a level of Pollution or Contaminates that are at, or below, the Safe level for Human consumption and is not a threat to our Health.

- Bad/Unsafe Water: Water that contains a level of Pollutants or Contaminates that is above the Safe level for Human consumption and may be a threat to our Health.

- Deadly Water: Water that contains a level of Pollution or Contaminates that is seriously above an Unsafe Level for Human consumption and subjects all living Creatures and Creation to these Deadly Waters.

Personal Water

I use three types of Water: Faucet, Filtered, and Bottled:

My Tap Water is for general purposes and has been treated as per our community in which it serves. I assume the quality is safe enough for general uses.

My Filtered Water is for cooking and rinsing off fruits and vegetables using countertop filtering. I assume the quality is safe for my intended use.

My Bottled Water is for drinking and mixing drinks, using Artesian Well Water. I assume it is safe for my intended use.

Having A Drink

For most of us who live in America, when we think of *having a drink*, what comes to the mind of many, is an alcoholic beverage; but for many people in other parts of the World, that might mean just a little sip of Life-Sustaining, Safe Water.

Relating to Water

Let's take a moment to reflect on Water. When God created Earth, Water was safe, readily available, and free to all the world;

but now has become unsafe, scarce, and costly to all the world. Something to think about.

Life Still Depends on It

In spite of all the Pollution and Contamination in Water, all Creatures and Creation still need and use it to sustain Life.

My Health and Wellness

Is

My Responsibility

To Drink The **Best Water** That I Can

CHAPTER 8

Hypertension Treatment – Air

Definition of Air

In the beginning, God Created the Heaven and Earth. Heaven was the space, or Atmosphere, above and around Earth. The Atmosphere, or air, that is made up of Nitrogen, Oxygen, and a few other gases is something we need to sustain Life.

Importance of Air

Air is one of the three essential components in the Physical Life-Sustaining trinity, along with Food and Water. Air has two of the same inherent characteristics that are a matter of Life or Death.

Company Air Keeps

Air, as with Food and Water, can contain Life-Sustaining substances, as well as Life-Threatening substances, such as Pollution and Contamination, that are in the Air we breathe.

The same Air that helps us to maintain good Health and Life, is the same Stuff that can adversely affect our Health and Life, when it is unsafe to Breathe.

Maintaining The Air

The Environmental Protection Agency, EPA; Occupational Safety & Health Administration, OSHA; U.S. Consumer Products Safety Commission; and other federal government agencies try to keep the public informed about the environments in which we work and live. All of these Agencies have serious concerns for safe levels of Air for the U.S. Population, both Outdoors and Indoors.

The agencies know many of the Pollutants that are in our Air, and know how to keep some of them within a safe level. But because there is so much Pollution and Con-tamination from so many different known and unknown sources, the agencies cannot always assure us that there are safe levels of Outdoor Air or Indoor Air for us humans to breathe.

Indoor Air

I think of my indoor quarters as my heav-en and earth, the ceiling as heaven, floor as earth. Everything between the floor and ceiling is my atmosphere, Air.

My living quarters being my universe, it is my Responsibility to maintain a good at-mospheric environment at all times, because every breath that I breathe to sustain Life, is within my little indoor universe.

The Indoor Air, what most Elderly and Shut-ins breathe most of the time, can be more threatening by more Pollutants than Outdoor Air. Many of these Pollutants are disguised by their cleaning power, by their hypnotic fragrances, and any other tech-nique that can be used to deceive and spread their poison. Some of these villains are common items on our regular shopping list:

- Laundry Products with artificial fragrances
- Deodorants
- Aftershave lotion
- Mouth wash
- Hair spray
- Carpet-Cleaning products
- Furniture Polish
- Plug-in Air Fresheners. One study found that more than fifteen different volatile organic compounds were emitted, seventeen regulated as toxic or hazardous under federal law.

<u>Personal Pollution</u>

Don't forget our personal contribution to Air Pollution. Each day we breathe about two pounds of Carbon Dioxide into the environment. All of us are regular contributors to Air Pollution, most noticeably Indoor Air.

Personal Contribution to Solution

- Acquire and use available knowledge on Indoor Air Pollution.

- Use an Air Filtering unit.

- Put Green Indoor House Plants throughout living unit. Pets also benefit.

- Vacuum carpet with a strong suction regularly.

- Use microfiber mops and dust cloths for dusting. They pick up more dust than the traditional fibers.

- Consider not smoking in your home. Cigarette smoke contains many harmful chemicals.

- Consider the harmful chemicals in commercial Air spray. I use an Essential Oil formula in a diffuser.

- Consider the harmful chemicals in commercial deodorants. I use an Essential Oil formula as deodorants.

- Consider the harmful chemicals in commercial aftershave lotion. I use an Essential Oil formula as aftershave lotion.

- Consider the harmful chemicals in commercial hair oil. I use an Essential Oil formula for hair and scalp.

- Consider harmful chemicals in commercial mouthwash. I use an Essential Oil formula for oral hygiene.

<u>Last Thought on Air</u>

The quality of your Health may depend on the quality of the Air you breathe. So I wish you well with your breathing.

My Health and Wellness

Is
My Responsibility

To Breathe The **<u>Best Air</u>** That I Can

CHAPTER 9

Hypertension Treatment – Exercise

<u>This is Exercise</u>

In this chapter, I will talk about Exercise as it relates to the Human Anatomy the Body, not the Mental or the Spiritual.

The definition or meaning of Physical Exercise is a routine of Bending the Joints, Flexing the Muscles, and putting Pressure on the Bones of the Human Anatomy. There are Routines and different Techniques that are followed to reach a particular objective.

There are two basic terms that are in play:

- **<u>Aerobic</u>**: This is the low-intensity Exercise that is in my Plan.

- **<u>Anaerobic</u>**: This is when you want to extend both the duration as well as the intensity of exercise.

Community At Work

There are three basic families of my Anatomy, that I want to be engaged in this community work. There are a whole bunch of these fellows in each of these three families:

- Joints
- Muscles
- Bones

Let's take a look at where these three families are going to be working, starting at the upper portion of my Anatomy and working down from my:

- Neck, Shoulders
- Arms, Elbows, Wrists, Hands, Fingers,
- Waist, Hips, Knees, Legs, Ankles, Feet, and Toes.

I stretch, flex, bend, and push the different Muscles, Joints, and Bones between my Neck and Toes using only my Body parts as equipment in performing all of my Techniques and Routines, doing whatever is necessary to get all the family members of the Anatomy involved.

When and How I Do It

I start some of my Exercise Routines in the morning in bed, on my Back. I do four Techniques while in bed that works as a good Exercise Primer.

After getting out of bed, and doing my Devotion, I do my Standing Routine Exercise. The movement of Oxygen to all the areas that are in motion is the definition of exercise. Having performed all of these Routines and Techniques, my whole Anatomy family have played a part.

During the day I will do some Sitting Routines, maybe while watching TV or listening to music.

My main event is the outdoor feature, my Walking Routine. This gave me a tremendous boost when I was starting my Hypertension Treatment.

The Same But Not as Much

- I still do my in-bed, on-Back Routines, putting in just as much time as before.

- Still doing my Standing Routines same as before.

- My Sitting Routines are not as often as before, because I am committed to some other things that use my Sitting time.

- My Walking Routine is reduced to about a distance of one-fourth of a mile per day, seven days per week. At the start of my Treatment, my Walking Routine was one mile per day four to five times per week. I continued that schedule until my Hypertension was under control, without the use of Medication.

<u>Something To Remember</u>

The Anatomy of the Human body was designed for Mobility, Exercise is necessary for it to maintain that Mobility;

If I don't give my Anatomy the Exercise it needs, then my Anatomy will not give me the Mobility I need.

My Health and Wellness

Is

My Responsibility

To Do The **Best Exercise** That I Can

CHAPTER 10

Hypertension Monitoring

<u>Defining Monitoring</u>

The word Monitor, or Monitoring, usually means to be aware of a situation or condition and of any changes that may take place within the confines of the situation or condition.

Defining the two-word term Hypertension Monitoring is a process. The word Monitor is, grammatically, a noun. But add ing, and the word becomes a participle. Join the word with Hypertension to form a two-word term, Hypertension Monitoring can be defined as a process that:

- Describes the details of the characteristics of the term and

- Explains the behavior, purpose and action of the term.

I acquired some decisive experience performing in-home Hypertension Monitoring during the years 2006 to 2010. By checking my Blood Pressure several times a day for many weeks and months, some days three times per day, was a routine that provided me a wealth of information.

The Monitoring information gave me an opportunity to act and react to every change in my blood pressure and observe responsiveness to different influences. It enabled me to make adjustments in different situations that influenced my Blood Pressure. I could see Hypertension Monitoring defining itself by displaying its characteristics in my ongoing interaction process.

Another very important thing I noticed about my Hypertension Monitoring is the ultra Sensitivity or Responsiveness to the environment in and outside the Body such as:

- Eating
- Drinking
- Exercising

- Bathing
- Low Or High Room Temperatures
- Looking At Scenes That Disturb Or Excite
- Loud Sounds
- Reading Serious Material
- Taxing The Mind By Fear Or Anxiety
- Thinking Unpleasant Thoughts
- Incorrect Posture
- Movements And Discomfort Of The Body
- Irregular Breathing

Effects Before, During, and After Activities

Before and during my Blood Pressure readings at my morning session, I would reflect on the night before:

- What Foods did I consume before bedtime, how much, if any?
- What activities before bedtime, how much, if any?
- What about my sleep; how much; was it quality?

Before and during my Blood Pressure readings at afternoon sessions, I would reflect on my morning and afternoon activities:

- What Foods did I consume for breakfast, and how much?

- What Foods did I consume for lunch, and how much, if any?

- What activities did I do before the afternoon session, and how much?

Before and during my Blood Pressure readings at my evening session, I would reflect on evening activities:

- What foods did I consume for dinner, how much?

- What snacks did I consume after dinner, how much, if any?

- What activities just before my session, how much, if any?

I was always consciously aware of the above activities and the influences before and during my Hypertension Monitoring sessions.

Later in the book, I will talk about the relative environmental areas inside and outside my Body, and how they relate to each other and my total person.

Regular Sessions

I did my Hypertension Monitoring regularly. In fact, I did three sessions daily at: 8:00 a.m, 2:00 p.m., and 8:00 p.m. I used three different Monitors during each session.

I took five Blood Pressure readings, three readings from one monitor, and one reading from each of the other two Monitors, each reading at intervals of five minutes.

The three different Monitors—two Cuff, and one Wrist type—provided me with an accuracy comparison of my Blood Pressure readings of Hypertension Monitoring.

Keeping in mind that my Blood Pressure and my Pulse Rate are subject to constant change. My Monitoring should be often, regular, and accurate, much like a security surveillance system. I didn't want to miss anything.

Remember, I was not monitoring Normal Blood Pressure, it was High Blood Pressure, Hypertension, so I took a very serious approach. My High Blood Pressure told my Monitor that something abnormal, or maybe serious, was happening somewhere within my body. In fact, it was possibly a Killer.

My Medical Instruments

Learning to use these Monitors correctly was very important to me, so I spent some time playing around with them, reading the manuals and carefully following the instructions.

These were my very own medical instruments that could give me the same information about my Blood Pressure—that my doctor provided—without having to visit my doctor's office.

One other medical instrument that I could call my own, a Temporal Thermometer, the type you swipe across your forehead and it shows a digital readout, let me know if I was running hot or cold.

Monitoring For Life

I took the time to take advantage of the invaluable information I was able to glean from the Blood Pressure readings, which related to different activities, and I could make changes and adjustments accordingly.

Keeping a log of all my Blood Pressure readings was very important. It provided a permanent history of my Blood Pressure all along the journey. Without Blood Pressure Monitoring, I could not have been able to navigate my journey.

My Health and Wellness

Is
My Responsibility

To do the **Best Monitoring** that I Can

CHAPTER 11

Hypertension Treatment Monitors

Need For A Monitor

These are my indispensable Medical Instruments, Blood Pressure Monitors. In fact, I have four of them—two Cuff types and two Wrist types. I shall never forget how useful they were during my Hypertension Treatment. They played a major role in doing what they were designed to do: read my Blood Pressure. I could not have followed my Treatment procedure without having the use of, at least one, in-home Blood Pressure Monitor.

A Special Place

In my bedroom, I have an older chest of drawers/desk combination. The top portion has a drop-down leaf that converts into a desk top. In the back portion of the desktop, there are shelves and a space for small office accessories.

I wanted to share this information with you about this place that, to me, is really *a Special Place*.

• This is where I display my Blood Pressure Monitors.

• This is where I perform all of my Monitoring sessions.

• This is where I display my Holy Bible.

• This is where I perform my daily Devotion.

• This is where I was reassured of having sufficient Knowledge, Faith, and Courage to carry out my Plan to Control and Cure my Primary Hypertension without the use of medication.

Monitors Roll Call

First Monitor is a Cuff-type Blood Pressure Monitor, comes with a Comfit Cuff, CD-ROM, USB Cable, AC Adapter, and 4 AA Batteries.

This unit uses the oscillometric method of Blood Pressure measurement. This means it detects the blood's movement through the brachial artery, and converts the movement into a digital reading. This unit stores measurement results for two people, A and B, listing Morning and Evening Averages. TruRead, another feature, allows for three consecutive measurements with timed intervals for an average reading.

The software included in this unit allows me to view, process, and print data about Blood Pressure and Pulse Rate measured by this unit. This is the first Monitor unit I use in my sessions, taking three initial readings at 5-minute intervals.

Second Monitor is a Wrist-type Blood Pressure Monitor, comes with a CD-ROM, Serial USB Cable, 2 AAA batteries, and a Storage Case. This unit uses the oscillometric method of Blood Pressure measurement. This means the unit detects the blood movement through the artery in the wrist and converts the movement into a digital reading.

The software included with this unit allows me to view, process, and print data about Blood Pressure and Pulse Rate measured by the unit, and upload this data to the computer. This is the second Monitor I use in my sessions. This unit has an Advanced Positioning Sensor that confirms that the unit is level with the my Heart, and this helps ensure that each reading is accurate and reliable.

Third Monitor is a Cuff-type Blood Pressure Monitor, comes with a Cuff, and 4 AA Batteries, and does not include any software. This unit uses the oscillometric method of Blood Pressure measurement. This means the unit detects your blood's movement through the brachial artery and converts the movement into a digital reading of Blood Pressure and Pulse Rate. This unit does not provide a memory feature to store the measurements. This is the third Monitor I use in my sessions.

Forth Monitor is a Wrist-type Blood Pressure Monitor, comes with 2 AAA Batteries, and a Storage Case. This unit uses the oscillometric method of Blood Pressure measurement. This means the unit detects my Blood's movement through the artery in my wrist and converts the movements into a digital reading of Blood Pressure and Pulse Rate, with a memory to store and recall the measurements.

This unit does not have the Advanced Positioning Sensor that confirms that the unit is level with my heart.

Body Temperature

Taking my Body temperature was always a part of my sessions. I used a Temporal Thermometer, an Infrared Temporal Scanner. This unit comes with a 9 volts Battery, and a plastic cap to cover the scanner head when not in use.

To get a Body Temperature reading, I press a little button on the front of the unit and do a gentle scan across my forehead and a digital Temperature appears in a little window on the face of the unit.

During all my sessions, I take and log three temperature readings; I wanted to be aware of my body temperature.

Qualities or Characteristics

I would like to believe that the qualities or characteristics of a Blood Pressure Monitor would be pretty much like some of the qualities or characteristics of a person: dependable, reliable, truthful, and accurate, because a life might depend on it.

> # My Health and Wellness
>
> Is
> My Responsibility
>
> To Use The **Best Monitors** That I Can

CHAPTER 12

Hypertension Treatment – Spirituality

Mind, Soul, Spirit

… Great is the Mystery of Godliness …
(I Timothy 3:16)

Christ, Alpha and Omega
Faith, Path to God
Word of God, Life
Revelation 1:8, 11; 21:6; 22:13

Spiritual Welcoming

At this time, I want to acknowledge and welcome my audience who might Believe and Practice one of the following Belief Systems:

- Agnostics, Persons denying God's existence is provable, or ones who believe that it is impossible to know whether or not God exists.

- Atheists, Persons who do not believe in God or deities.

- Buddhists, Persons who practice Buddhism, a world religion or philosophy based on the teaching of the Buddha and holding that a state of enlightenment can be attained by suppressing worldly desires.

- Devils, who believe there *is*, but not *in* God, and tremble!

- Fools, who believe there is no God.

- Hindus, Persons who practice the religion of Hinduism, the religion of India, and the oldest of the worldwide religions, character-ized by a belief in reincarnation.

- Jews, Persons who are Believers in Judaism, members of a Semitic People, descendants from the ancient Hebrews who recorded, for the world, the Holy Scriptures. The Scriptures include two of the most recog-nizable Titles: God's Ten Commandments (Exodus 20:3-17), (Deuteronomy 5:7-21), and Psalm 23.

- Muslims, Persons who Believe in and Practice Islam.

- Others not mentioned, Persons of other beliefs and practices.

- Christians, Persons who Believe and Practice the Gospel of Jesus Christ as taught in the Holy Bible, Holy Scriptures, Inspired Word of God. This includes:

  A. Persons who Believe that there is One God, Three Entities: Father, Son, and Holy Spirit.

  B. Persons who Believe that all persons are born with a sinful Nature, the same Nature as Adam's, after the Fall.

  C. Persons who Believe, "If you confess with your mouth, the Lord Jesus, and Believe in your Heart that God raised Him from the dead, you shall be Saved; for with your Heart , you Believe unto Righteousness, and with your mouth Confession is made unto Salvation." (Romans 10:9-10). Unless a person is Spiritually born again, he or she cannot see and understand the Spiritual things of God, from Faith to Faith.

D. Persons who Believe that "God so Loved the world, that He gave His Only Begotten Son, and whosoever believes in Him, should not perish, but have everlasting Life". John 3:16)

E. Persons who Believe God was Manifested or Revealed in the flesh. (I Timothy 3:16)

F. Persons who have accepted Jesus Christ, and are Heirs of God and Joint-Heirs with Christ. (Romans 8:17)

G. Persons who Believe that Christ, the Son of God, came to this world, suffered, and died on the Cross for our sins, and was raised from the dead for our Justification. (1 Timothy 1:15), (Romans 4:25)

H. Persons who Believe that the Gospel of Jesus Christ is the Power of God to Salvation for everyone who Believes, for the Jews and also for the Gentiles. (Romans 1:16)

I. Persons who Believe that in the Gospel of Christ, the Righteousness of God is revealed from Faith to Faith. (Romans 1:17)

J. Persons who Believe we walk by Faith. (II Corinthians 5:7)

K. Persons who Believe that Faith is the Substance of Things Hoped for and the Evidence of Things not Seen. (Hebrews 11:1)

L. Persons who can legally claim all the Rights and Benefits in God's Plan of Salvation, which includes Healing and Curing of Diseases and Illnesses. (Psalms 107:20), (Isaiah 53:5),(Matthew 10:1), (I Peter 2:24)

M. Persons who Believe that the whole World is Guilty before God. (Romans 3:19)

Spiritual Procedures

In Spiritual Procedures, we start with Spiritual Guidelines; and those Guidelines are found in the Holy Bible, the Inspired Word of God.

The Holy Bible in the Natural is just a book. But in the Spiritual, it is the Book of books, and as God has told others in His Book, He tells me basically the same thing, "If I will observe to do all that is written in His Holy Book, then I will prosper and be successful in all that concerns me, including Body, Mind, Soul, and Spirit." (Joshua 1:8)

Word Of God

The Word of God has been on display since the Creation of the World, so there is no excuse for me to not have more knowledge of His Word. As I learn more about God's Word, I will understand the real meaning of "He Is As Good As His Word." But until I was born again by the Word of God and the Spirit of God, I could not experience that understanding.

God has given us a few Words, in His Word. The meaning of His Word:

"The Word of God is Life, and Powerful, and Sharper than any Two-Edged Sword, Piercing even to the dividing asunder of Soul and Spirit, and of the Joints and Marrow, and is a Discerner of the Thoughts and Intents of the Heart." (Hebrews 4:12)

Living The Spiritual Experiences

In the previous chapters I shared with you my experiences on how I sustained my Physical Life, and how I nourish my Physical Body with the best available Physical Food, Water, and Air, which are three-fourths of _What I am._

In this chapter, I will share with you my experiences on how I sustain my Spiritual Life by nourishing it with the best available Spiritual Food, which is the other one-fourth of _what I am_, and also _who I am._

The Equation:

Physical		Spiritual		what and
				who I am
Three-fourth	plus	one-fourth	equal	four-fourth
3/4	+	1/4	=	4/4

The Two Natures

God Made man from the dust of the Earth; but He Created man from His Spirit. Remember, the part of man He Made is (_what I am_) Natural, Physical, and Earthy; and the part of man He Created is (_who I am_) Spiritual, and in His Likeness. (Genesis 1:26-27; 2:7)

Spiritual Nourishment

In chapter six, I presented the Physical aspects of my Menu:

- What I eat: Food
- What I drink: Water
- What I breathe: Air

All of these elements are essential to sustain Physical life And now I'll discuss the Spiritual Life.

Spiritual Life; Faith and Christ

To sustain my Spiritual Life, Spiritual Food, which is the Word of God, it is essential to grow in Grace, and the Knowledge of our Lord Jesus Christ. This Spiritual Food benefits my Spiritual Life only through the Faith of Christ. (I Peter 2:2), (II Peter 3:18)

Without the Faith of Christ, it is impossible to please God. It is impossible to understand the things of God, it is impossible to grow Spiritually (Hebrews 11:6),(II Peter1:5-10). Since the Faith of Christ is essential to my

Spiritual Life, let's look at the meaning of Faith:

"Faith Is the Substance of Things Hoped for, and Is the Evidence of things not seen." (Hebrews 11:1)

The meaning of Faith has Christ as the Author and Finisher. He Is the Substance. He is the Evidence. He *is* Faith Personified, and the Alpha and Omega. (Hebrews 12:2), (Revelation 1:8,11)

<u>Baby Food</u>

After my Spiritual Birth, as it was after my Natural birth, I had to learn to walk. As a newborn Babe in Christ, I had to learn to walk by Faith.

All babies desire milk. Spiritual babies desire the sincere milk of the Word of God that they might grow in Faith. (I Peter 2:2)

By hearing and reading the Word of God from the Holy Bible, their Faith increases and they grow in Grace and Knowledge of Jesus Christ, Who Is also the Object of their Faith. (Romans 10:17)

Relationships in the Cycle of Life

- In the Natural, Food nutrients flow in the Blood .

- In the Spiritual, Food nutrients flow in Faith.

- In the Natural, Life flows in the Blood.

- In the Spiritual, Life flows in Faith.

When we think of relationships, it is usually in reference to an affiliation, association, or a friendship with someone or others. But there are relationships within both the Natural Anatomy and the Spiritual Anatomy:

- In the Natural, the Brain relates to the Nerves. The Nerves relate to the brain, the Nerves relate to the Body Anatomy. The Body Anatomy relates to the Nerves. The Body Anatomy reacts or responds to the activities of the Nerves and Manifestation takes place in some part or parts of the Body Anatomy, as either Sickness, Disease, Death or Health and Wellness. Then Back to the Brain in the reverse order, a Systemic Process.

- In the Spiritual, the Mind relates to the Brain, and the Brain relates to the Mind. The Mind relates to the Soul, and the Soul relates to the Mind. The Soul relates to the Spirit, and the Spirit relates to the Soul. The Spirit relates to God, and God, the Father, relates to the Son. The Son relates to the Spirit, and the Godhead reacts. Then Back to the Natural by way of Spirit, Soul, Mind, Brain, Nerves, and Body Anatomy . Then these things react or respond to the activities of the Nerves and Manifestation takes place in some part or parts of the Body Anatomy as Health and Wellness. Then Back to the Mind in the reverse order, a Systemic Process.

<u>Growing in Grace and Knowledge</u>

My Spiritual Birth has taken place, I have nurtured and grown on the milk of God's Word, now walking by Faith and ready to work out God's Plan of Salvation that I inherited at the time when I accepted the Gospel of Christ. The Gospel of Christ is the Birth,

Life, Death, Burial, and Resurrection of Christ, which is the Gospel of Himself. (Romans 1:16), (Philippians 2:12-13)

In the Gospel of Christ, is the Power of God that provides me His Plan of Salvation. His plan includes a whole bunch of Gifts that I can open and enjoy each and every day of this Life and into Life after this Life.

Here are some of the Gifts in this Spiritual Package: Spiritual Vitamins and Supplements, some of God's priceless Blessings:

A. Brotherly Kindness

B. Courage

C. Deliverance

D. Eternal Life

E. Faith

F. Forgiveness

G. Glorification

H. Grace

I. Healing

J. Justification

K. Knowledge

L. Love

M. Obedience

N. Patience

O. Power

P. Perseverance

Q. Redemption

R. Righteousness

S. Sanctification

T. Temperance

U. Virtue

V. Wisdom

These Blessings are mine, on which to think and meditate day and night. The Power of the Holy Spirit helps me grow into the Manifestation of all the above and More. (II Peter 3:18)

DAILY DEVOTION

Prayer and Scripture Reading

Morning Prayer

All parts of this Prayer are memorized passages of the Word of God, I pray before getting out of bed:

- _Thanking My Father_

"Holy Father, I thank You for another day. I present my body as a living sacrifice, Holy and acceptable to You, which is my reasonable service. Help me in the process of renewing of my mind, that I might be able to prove what is that Good, Acceptable, and the Perfect Will of God. (Romans 12:1-2)

I wash my hands and my feet to remove any residual sins from working and walking in this World. I will feast on the Show bread, which is the Body of Christ under the Power and light of Your Holy Spirit.

I approach Your Throng of Grace to Petition, Intercede, Praise and give Thanks. I give Thanks first of all for Jesus Christ, Your Holy Spirit, and Your Word. Thank You for Blessing all of Your Saints, all of their family members, all of your Creatures, and I Praise You for Your Creation."

- *Renewing My Mind*

"Thank you for the renewing of my mind, that I am to think on things that are True, Honest, Just and Pure, and whatsoever things that are Lovely and if there be any Praise help me to think on these things. (Philippians 4:8)

And Lord, help me to add to my Faith, Virtue and to Virtue, Knowledge and to Knowledge, Temperance,; and to Temperance, Patience and to Patience, Godliness; and to Godliness, Brotherly Kindness; and to Brotherly Kindness, Charity, which is Love." (II Peter 1:5-7)

- *The Lord, Who Blesses Me*

"Bless the Lord, oh my Soul and all that is within me,. Bless His Holy Name,. Bless the Lord,

oh my Soul and forget not all His Benefits It is He Who Forgives all my iniquities, Who Heals all my Diseases, Who Redeems my Life from Destruction, Who Crowns me with Lovely Kindness and Tender Mercies Who Satisfies my Mouth with Good Things, That my Youth be Renewed as the Eagle's."(Psalms 103:1-5)

- *My Shepherd*

"The Lord is my Shepherd, I shall not want. He makes me to lie down in green pastures, He leads me besides the still Waters. He restores my Soul. He leads me in the path of Righteousness for His Name's Sake.

Yea, though I walk through the Valley of the Shadow of Death, I will fear no evil, for You are with me. Your Rod and Your Staff, They Comfort me. You prepared a Table for me in the presence of my enemies. You have anointed my head with Oil, my cup runs over. Surely Goodness and Mercy shall follow me all the days of my Life, and I will dwell in the House of the Lord, Forever." (Psalms 23:1-6)

- *Love Note*

"Though I speak with the Tongues of Men and of Angels, and have not Charity, I am nothing. Though I have the Gift of Prophecy, and Understand all Mysteries and all Knowledge, and have all Faith, that I could remove mountains, and have not Charity, I am nothing.

Though I bestow all my goods to feed the poor, and though, I present my Body to be burned, and have not Charity, it profits me nothing. Charity suffers long and is Kind. Charity does not envy. Charity does not boast. It is not puffed up, does not behave Itself unseemly. It seeks not Her own, and is not easily provoked. It thinks no evil and Rejoices not in iniquity, but Rejoices in the Truth. It bears all things, Believes all Things, Hopes all Things, and endures all things.

Charity never fails, but if there be Prophecies, they shall fail. If there be Tongues, they shall cease. If there be Knowledge, it shall vanish away. For we know in part, and we Prophecy in part, but when that which is Perfect is come, then all that is in part shall be done away.

When I was child, I spoke as a child. I understood as a child, I thought as a child. But when I became a man, I put away childish things. Now we see through a glass darkly, but then face to face. Now I know in part, but then shall I know even as also I am known. Now abides Faith, Hope, Charity, these three, but the greatest of these is Charity."
(I Corinthians 13:1-13)

- *Wickedness in the World*

"The wrath of God is revealed from Heaven against all ungodliness and unrighteousness of men who suppress the Truth in unrighteousness. That which may be known of God is manifested in them, for God has shown it to them. For the invisible things of God from the Creation of the World are clearly seen. Being understood by the things that are made, even His Eternal Power and Godhead, so they are without excuse.

Because of that, when they knew God, they glorified Him not as God, neither were they thankful, but became vain in their imaginations, and their foolish hearts were darkened. Professing to be wise, they became fools, and changed the Glory of the incorruptible God into an image made like a corruptible man, and to birds, and four-footed beasts, and creeping things.

Therefore, God also gave them up to uncleanness through the lusts of their own hearts, to dishonor their own bodies between themselves, who changed the Truth of God into a lie, and worshiped and served the creature more than the Creator, Who is Blessed forever. Amen.

For this cause, God gave them up unto vile affections, for even their women changed the natural use into that which is against Nature. And, likewise, also the men leaving the natural use of the woman, burned in their lust one toward another, men with men working that which is unseemly, and receiving in themselves that recompense of their error which was due.

And even as they did not like to retain God in their knowledge, God gave them over to a debased mind, to do those things which are not fitting, being filled with all unrighteousness, sexual immorality, wickedness, covetousness, maliciousness, full of envy, murder, strife, deceit, evil mindedness, whisperers, backbiters, haters of God, violent, proud, boasters, inventors of evil things, disobedient to parents, undiscerning, untrustworthy, unloving, unforgiving, and unmerciful.

Who, knowing the righteous judgment of God, that those who practice such things are deserving of death, not only do the same, but also approve of those who practice them." (Romans 1:18-32)

- *Ready For Daily Battle*

"Lord help me to remember that I have '... the whole Armour of God that I might be able to stand against the wiles of the devil. And remember that I am not fighting against flesh and blood, but against Powers, Principalities, against the rulers of darkness, against Spiritual wickedness in High Places.

And help me remember that I need the whole Armour of God, that I might stand in the evil day. And having done all, to stand, having my Loins girt with Truth, and having on the Breastplate of

Righteousness, and my feet shod with the Prepara-tion of the Gospel of Peace.

And above all, having the Shield of Faith, that I shall be able to quench all the fiery darts of the wicked. And wearing the Helmet of Salvation, and having the Sword of the Spirit, which is the Word of God. And Praying always with Prayer and Sup-plication in the Spirit, and watching with all Per-severance and Supplication for all the Saints.'" *(Ephesians 6:11-18)*

• *Benediction*

"Lord, show me the path in which I should walk, knowing that in that path are Mercy and Truth, and that in Your Presence is Fullness of Joy, and at Your Right Hand are Pleasures Forevermore! (Psalm 16:11)

Now unto You, Who is able to do Exceeding, Abundantly above All that I ask or think Accord-ing to the Power that works within me, Glory to God. (Ephesians 3:20)

Now. unto You, Who is able to keep me from falling, and to present me faultless before the

Presence of Your Glory, with Exceeding Joy To the Only Wise God, my Savior, be Glory and Majesty, Dominion and Power, both now and ever. Amen."
(Jude 24-25)

- *Morning Scripture Reading*

After my Morning Prayer and I am out of bed, I read two or three chapters of Scripture in the Old Testament and one chapter in the New Testament of the Holy Bible. This daily schedule takes me through the entire Bible in one year.

<u>Evening Prayer</u>

I usually pray my evening prayer when I am taking my bath. While relaxing in my tub of nice, warm water, I pray most of my morning Prayer.

Conclusion

It has been a pleasure sharing with you, my experience and testimony of the Natural and Spiritual procedures of my Alternative Treatment for Hypertension Control and Cure without Medication. I hope that you may experience the personal Responsibility to do the best that you can to obtain and maintain your Health and Wellness.

My Health and Wellness

Is
My Responsibility

To Know, Trust, And Obey God's Word

So Be It, Amen

ABOUT THE AUTHOR

The author of this book is an Intermediate Elderly man who lives alone with four indoor green plants, two computers: a laptop, and a desktop. on which he spends much of his time. His serious interests are; Spirituality, Health, children, grand children, and great grand children. His casual interests are chess, table tennis, old movies, and jazz music.

For more of my personal aspects of Hypertension, visit: www.hypertension-control-cure.com

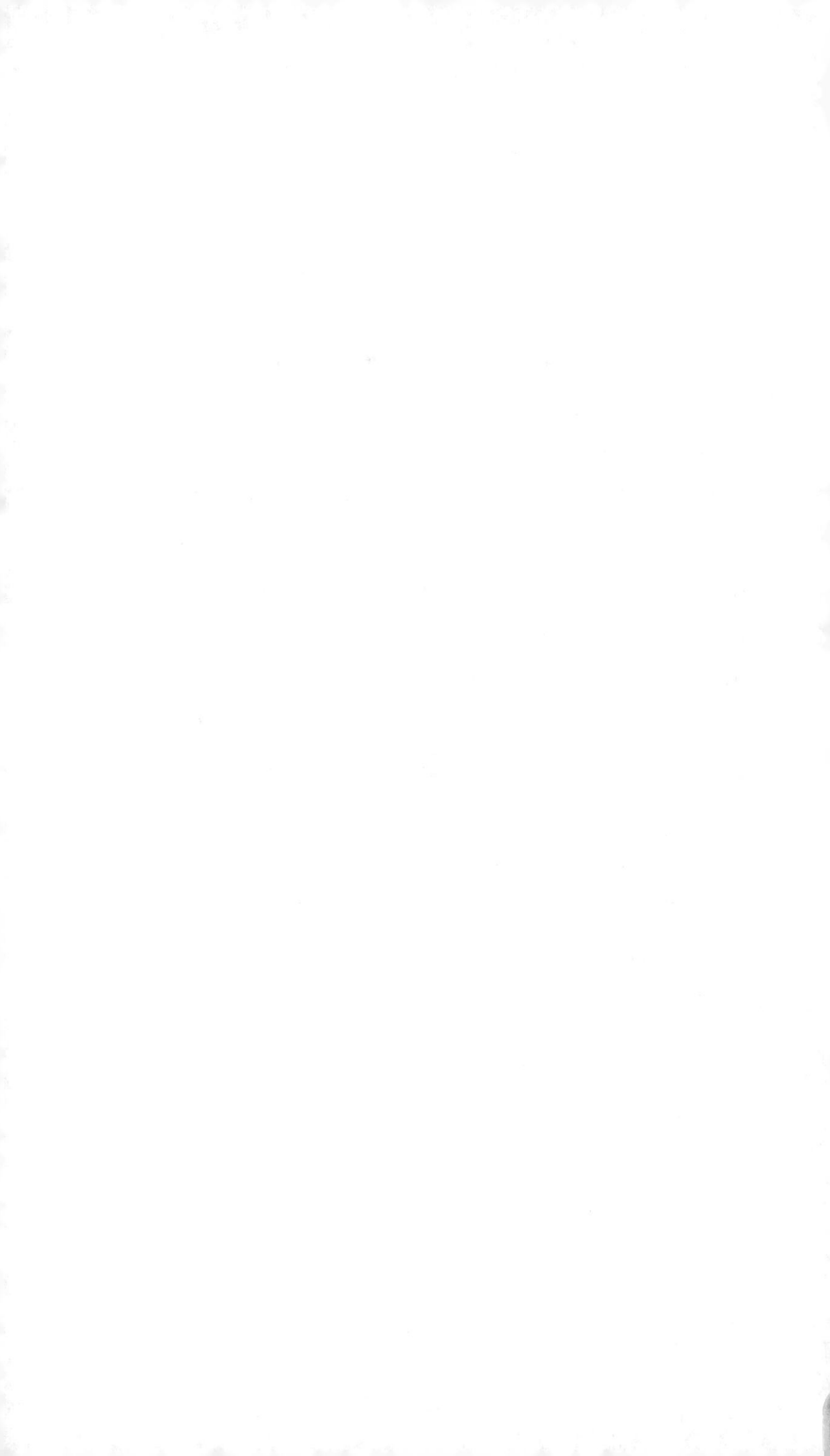

www.ingramcontent.com/pod-product-compliance
Lightning Source LLC
Chambersburg PA
CBHW070151290526
45789CB00002B/718